Healthy Vegetarian

A Perfectly Crafted Guide in Becoming a Healthy Vegetarian

Chinaza Precious Silvanous

DEDICATION

This Book is Dedicated to my Mom, Friends and to those who have not found my content yet.

CONTENTS

Chapter 1

Introduction

Chapter 2

Educate Yourself

Chapter 3

Gradual Transition

Chapter 4

Diverse and Balanced Diet

Chapter 5

Protein-Rich Plant Foods

Chapter 6

Monitor Nutrient Intake

Chapter 7

Embrace Whole Foods

Chapter 8

Explore Plant-Based Alternatives

Chapter 9
Stay Hydrated

Chapter 10
Listen to Your Body

Chapter 11
Conclusion

CHAPTER 1

Adopting a vegetarian lifestyle can be a transformative journey for both your health and the environment. Whether you're motivated by ethical, environmental, or health reasons, making the switch to a vegetarian diet requires careful consideration and planning. This guide aims to provide you with a roadmap to becoming a healthy vegetarian, ensuring that you meet your nutritional needs while enjoying a diverse and

DELICIOUS ARRAY OF PLANT-BASED FOODS.

DELICIOUS ARRAY OF PLANT-BASED FOODS.

CHAPTER 2

EDUCATE YOURSELF:

BEFORE EMBARKING ON YOUR VEGETARIAN JOURNEY, IT'S ESSENTIAL TO EDUCATE YOURSELF ABOUT THE NUTRITIONAL REQUIREMENTS OF A PLANT-BASED DIET. **U**NDERSTANDING THE KEY NUTRIENTS FOUND IN VARIOUS PLANT FOODS AND HOW TO COMBINE THEM FOR OPTIMAL HEALTH IS CRUCIAL. **K**EY NUTRIENTS INCLUDE PROTEIN,

IRON, CALCIUM, VITAMIN B12, OMEGA-3 FATTY ACIDS, AND ZINC.

CHAPTER 3

Gradual Transition:

Transitioning to a vegetarian lifestyle doesn't have to happen overnight. Consider taking gradual steps, such as starting with meatless Mondays or incorporating more plant-based meals into your diet. This approach allows your taste buds and digestive system to adjust gradually.

CHAPTER 4

Diverse and Balanced Diet:

A well-balanced vegetarian diet includes a variety of fruits, vegetables, whole grains, legumes, nuts, and seeds. Aim for a colorful plate to ensure you're getting a diverse range of nutrients. Experiment with different cuisines and cooking methods to keep your meals exciting and satisfying.

CHAPTER 5

Protein-Rich Plant Foods:

Protein is a crucial component of any diet, and it's readily available in plant-based sources. Incorporate protein-rich foods like beans, lentils, tofu, tempeh, quinoa, and edamame into your meals. Combining different plant protein sources throughout the day can ensure you meet

your protein needs.

CHAPTER 6

Monitor Nutrient Intake:

Keep an eye on your nutrient intake, especially for nutrients that are more challenging to obtain from a vegetarian diet, such as vitamin B12 and omega-3 fatty acids. Consider fortified foods or supplements if needed, but consult with a healthcare professional to ensure you're meeting your nutritional requirements.

CHAPTER 7

Embrace Whole Foods:

Opt for whole, minimally processed foods as the foundation of your vegetarian diet. Whole grains, fruits, vegetables, and legumes provide essential nutrients and fiber, promoting overall health

and well-being.

CHAPTER 8

Explore Plant-Based Alternatives:

As the popularity of vegetarianism grows, so does the availability of plant-based alternatives to traditional animal products. Explore plant-based meat substitutes, dairy alternatives, and egg replacers to find products that suit your taste and nutritional preferences.

CHAPTER 9

Don't forget the importance of staying hydrated. Water is essential for overall health and can help you feel more satisfied between meals. Herbal teas and infused water are excellent choices to add variety to your hydration routine.

CHAPTER 10

Pay attention to your body's signals and adjust your diet accordingly. If you feel fatigued or notice any deficiencies, consult with a healthcare professional or a registered dietitian who specializes in vegetarian nutrition.

Conclusion: Becoming a healthy vegetarian is a rewarding and fulfilling journey that involves thoughtful planning and a commitment to a diverse, balanced diet. By educating yourself, making gradual changes, and embracing a variety of plant-based foods, you can enjoy the numerous health benefits that a vegetarian lifestyle has to offer while contributing to a more sustainable and compassionate world.

ABOUT THE AUTHOR

Chinaza Precious Silvanous is an expert when it comes to Healthy Vegetables for weight loss. She has used it and it worked wonders for her and is dedicated to helping others like yourself find the same measures of a perfect healthy diet.

One thing that makes this Book unique is that everything inside are from personal experience.